Copyright © 2019 by Emily green RND

All rights reserved. No part of this publication may be reproduced, distributed, or transmitted in any form or by any means, including photocopying, recording, or other electronic or mechanical methods, without the prior written permission of the publisher, except in the case of brief quotations embodied in critical reviews and certain other noncommercial uses permitted by copyright law

Table of Contents

INTRODUCTION 4

What is Diabetes 6

Diabetes epidemiology 6

Types of diabetes 7

Symptoms of diabetes 9

What happens in diabetes 10

Prevention, treatment and care 10

What Causes Diabetes? 11

Diabetes Diagnosis 16

Insulin treatment for diabetes 19

Types of insulin 19

Which insulin is best 24

How is insulin taken 25

Insulin delivery devices 26

Insulin plant for diabetes 33

Insulin Plant (Costus igneus) 33

Medicinal use 36

Health Benefits Of Insulin Plant 37

How Insulin Plant Cures Diabetes 45

How To Recognize Insulin Plant 46

From Where This Magical Herb Can Be Sourced 47

Different Names Of Insulin Plant 47

How to use Insulin plant to cure diabetes – DIY 48
Nutrition information 49
How to make insulin leaves raita 49
Recipe Notes 51
Research evidence 52
How To Consume Insulin Plant To Cure Diabetes- 53
How To Make Insulin Leaves Steeping 55
How To Make Tea Of Insulin Leaves 56
Final Talk 57

INTRODUCTION

About a year back, a wonderful local herbalist asked me whether I wanted to see a herb called insulin plant. Nothing makes me more happy than getting to know new herbs and when I nodded my head in agreement he took me to his backyard and showed me the insulin plant. I still remember staring at the plant mesmerized as the herbalist explained it's wonderful benefits and medicinal uses especially for diabetic patients.

Insulin plant is an Medicinal Herbal Plant It's a Magic Cure for Diabetes . It's leaf helps to build up insulin in the human body so it is commonly known as insulin plant in India .Insulin plant was grown in America and is becoming popular in India because of it's medicinal chemicals . It is now accepted and used widely as an Ayurvedic medicinal herb. Insulin plant belongs to the family Costaceae. Consumption of the leaves are believed to lower blood glucose levels, and diabetics who consumed the leaves of this plant did report a fall in their blood glucose levels.

Insulin plant is widely called in Malyalam "insulin chedi, where chedy means a plant. The catchphrase of this plant is " a leaf a day keeps diabetes away".

The plant is characterized by large fleshy looking leaves. It grows very quickly. Propagation is by stem cutting. It grows in slightly shady areas.

Diabetes Patients are advised to chew down a leaf in the morning and one in the evening for a month. Allopathic doctors too recommend it and it is found to be effective in bringing blood sugar levels under completely under control. There is also dried and ground powder of the leaves now available in the market.

This medicine is being increasingly prescribed by doctors. In 90 % of the cases diabetes has been found to be curable using this medicine. Just try it for yourself.

What is Diabetes

Diabetes is a condition where the body fails to utilize the ingested glucose properly. This could be due to lack of the hormone insulin or because the insulin that is available is not working effectively.

Diabetes mellitus

The term diabetes is the shortened version of the full name diabetes mellitus. Diabetes mellitus is derived from the Greek word diabetes meaning siphon - to pass through the Latin word mellitus meaning honeyed or sweet.This is because in diabetes excess sugar is found in blood as well as the urine. It was known in the 17th century as the "pissing evil".

Diabetes epidemiology

Diabetes is the fastest growing long term disease that affects millions of people worldwide. According to the charity Diabetes UK, more than two million people in the UK have the condition and up to 750,000 more are unaware of having the condition.

In the United States 25.8 million people or 8.3% of the population have diabetes. Of these, 7.0 million have undiagnosed diabetes. In 2010, about 1.9 million new cases of diabetes were diagnosed in population over 20 years. It is said that if this trend continues, 1 in 3 Americans would be diabetic by 2050.

Types of diabetes

There are two types of diabetes – Type 1 and type 2. Type 1 diabetes is called insulin-dependent diabetes mellitus and occurs at a younger age or childhood. In these patients there is complete lack of the hormone insulin that mandates external administration of the hormone regularly as treatment.

Around 75% of people with diabetes have type 2 diabetes mellitus. This was earlier termed non-insulin dependent diabetes mellitus (NIDDM) or maturity-onset diabetes mellitus. The number of people with type 2 diabetes is rapidly increasing. In type 2 diabetes, not enough insulin is produced or the insulin that is made by the body is insufficient to meet the needs of the body. Obesity or being overweight predisposes to type 2 diabetes.

Gestational diabetes

Gestational diabetes occurs in pregnant women who have never had diabetes before but who have high blood sugar levels during pregnancy. Gestational diabetes affects about 4% of all pregnant women. After childbirth the mother may go on to develop type 2 diabetes.

How is blood sugar regulated normally?

When food is taken, it is broken down to smaller components. Sugars and carbohydrates are thus broken down into glucose for the body to utilize them as energy source. The liver is also able to manufacture glucose.

In normal persons the hormone insulin, which is made by the beta cells of the pancreas, regulates how much glucose is in the blood. When there is excess glucose in the blood, insulin stimulates cells to absorb enough glucose from the blood for the energy that they need. Insulin also stimulates the liver to absorb and store any glucose that is excess in blood. Insulin release is triggered after a meal when there is rise in blood glucose. When blood glucose levels fall, during exercise for example, insulin levels fall too. A second hormone manufactured by the pancreas is called glucagon. It has the opposite function of stimulating the liver to release glucose when necessary.

Symptoms of diabetes

The main symptoms of diabetes are three – polydipsia, polyphagia and polyuria. These mean increased thirst, increased hunger and increased frequency of urination. In addition patients complain of feeling very tired and weight loss and loss of muscle bulk. Type 1 diabetes can develop quickly, over weeks or even days whereas type 2 diabetes may develop gradually.

What happens in diabetes

Due to lack or insufficiency of insulin there is high blood glucose in diabetes. Excess glucose in the blood can damage the blood vessels. This leads to several complications like heart disease, kidney damage, nerve damage, eye damage and blindness, impotence and stroke.

Diabetes, when not controlled, may raise the propensity for infections. Infections and gangrene of the lower limbs is common in uncontrolled diabetes. This may necessitate an amputation if severe. People with diabetes are also 15 per cent more likely to have an amputation than people without the condition.

Prevention, treatment and care

The risk of complications with diabetes can be reduced by adhering to medical advice and keeping diabetes under control. Blood sugar should be regularly monitored so that any problems can be detected and treated early.

Treatment involves both healthy diet and exercise as well as oral medications to regulate blood sugar. In all type 1 diabetics and in severe uncontrolled type 2 diabetics one or more injections of insulin a day may be needed.

What Causes Diabetes?

Diabetes mellitus results mainly from a deficiency or diminished effectiveness of insulin that is normally produced by the beta cells of the pancreas. It is characterised by high blood sugar, altered sugar and glucose metabolism and this affects blood vessels and causes several organ damage. Causes of diabetes can be classified according to the types of diabetes.

Type 1 diabetes mellitus

This results from the body's failure to produce sufficient insulin. Here the pancreatic beta cells are irreversibly damaged and so they cannot produce adequate insulin. This is believed to be due to an over active immune system that instead of fighting foreign microbes turns on the body's own cells and begins to destroy the pancreatic cells.

Since type 1 diabetes has been found in both identical twins in studies, four genes are thought to be important. One (6q) determines the sensitivity of the islet cells of pancreas to damage. This damage could be due to viruses or cross-reactivity from cow's milk-induced antibodies.

In addition, associations with HLA DR3 and DR4 and islet cell antibodies around the time of diagnosis have been noted. Risks of developing type 1 diabetes are similar in all ethnic groups. This could be due to diet during childhood or due to genes.

Type 2 diabetes mellitus

Type 2 diabetes mellitus results from a resistance to the insulin. There may be a normal or increased level of insulin initially. The pancreatic beta cells try to secrete more insulin initially to meet the raised demands of the body. When it fails, type 2 diabetes develops.

Risks for type 2 diabetes mellitus include excess body weight and physical inactivity. All racial groups are affected but increased prevalence in people of South Asian, African, African-Caribbean, Polynesian, Middle-Eastern and American-Indian ancestry is noted.

Other risk factors for type 2 diabetes include history of gestational diabetes, impaired glucose tolerance, impaired fasting glucose, drug use like thiazide diuretic along with a beta-blocker, low-fibre, high-glycaemic index diet, metabolic syndrome, Polycystic ovarian syndrome, family history and those who have a history of a low birth weight.

Gestational or pregnancy associated diabetes

Pregnant women who have never had diabetes before may develop increased demands for insulin during pregnancy. This may not be met by a raised insulin secretion and gestational diabetes results. This affects 4 to 5% of all pregnant women. It may precede development of type 2 (or rarely type 1) diabetes.

Maturity onset diabetes of the young

This is a combination of several forms of diabetes all resulting from a single genetic defect affecting the beta-cell function resulting in impaired insulin secretion. There may be slight high blood sugar at a young age. This genetic defect is usually inherited in an autosomal-dominant manner.

Secondary diabetes

Secondary diabetes occurs due to a disease affecting the pancreas or other endocrine organs. This accounts for 1 to 2% of all diabetics. Some of the causes of secondary diabetes include:- Diseases of the pancreas that may affect the beta cells – this includes cystic fibrosis, chronic pancreatitis, after surgical removal of the pancreas or due to pancreas cancer.

Diseases of the hormonal system of endocrine system – Cushing's syndrome (affecting adrenal glands), acromegaly (affecting the pituitary gland), thryrotoxicosis (excessive activity of the thyroid gland), peochromocytoma (affecting adrenal glands), glucagonoma (affecting glucagon producing cells of the pancreas).

Due to intake of certain drugs over long term - this includes water pills or diuretics like thiazides, corticosteroids, atypical antipsychotics, protease inhibitors used in HIV infection. Patients with Congenital lipodystrophy, Acanthosis nigricans etc. Those with genetic conditions like Wolfram syndrome also known as DIDMOAD standing for diabetes insipidus, diabetes mellitus, optic atrophy and deafness. Other genetic conditions predisposing to diabetes include Friedreich's ataxia, dystrophia myotonica, haemochromatosis, glycogen storage diseases etc.

Diabetes Diagnosis

Diabetes is diagnosed by performing a blood test. The test usually reveals high blood glucose. Steps in diagnosis includes:

If a patient presents with symptoms of diabetes a blood test for blood glucose is ordered. In most cases of type 2 diabetes mellitus there may be little or no symptoms. This means high blood sugar may be detected on a routine blood tests for example one taken before a surgery. It is important to make the diagnosis early since uncontrolled high blood glucose for a long duration leads to long term damage to blood vessels and other complications.

Diabetes is diagnosed on the basis of a single abnormal plasma glucose reading. When taken randomly at any time of the day the levels are significant if they are above 11.1 mmol/L and when taken after an overnight fast, the numbers are significant if above 7 mmol/L (126 mg/dL). This is considered positive for diabetes when there is presence of diabetic symptoms such as thirst, increased urination, recurrent infections, weight loss, drowsiness etc.

In people who have no symptoms an abnormal random plasma glucose followed by two more abnormal fasting blood glucose readings (over 7 mmol/L) is significant. Patients with fasting glucose levels from 100 to 125 mg/dL (6.1 and 7.0 mmol/L) are considered to have impaired fasting glucose.

Once an abnormal fasting blood glucose is obtained, blood glucose is tested again two hours after a full meal. This usually means after 75 g anhydrous glucose when an oral glucose tolerance test (OGTT) is performed. Readings over 11.1 mol/L is significant for diabetes. Patients with plasma glucose at or above 140 mg/dL or 7.8 mmol/L, but not over 200, two hours after a 75 g oral glucose load are considered to have impaired glucose tolerance. This raises the risk of acquiring diabetes in near future if uncontrolled.

The World Health Organization (WHO) now recommends that glycated haemoglobin (HbA1c) can be used as a diagnostic test for diabetes. This indicates the blood sugar control in an individual over the last three months. Even a single episode of uncontrolled blood sugar during this period can be detected as a high HbA1c. An HbA1c of 48 mmol/mol (6.5%) is the cut-off point for diagnosing diabetes. A value less than 6.5% does not however exclude diabetes diagnosed using blood glucose tests.

Diagnosis also involves assessment of damage to kidneys, eyes and other organs due to long standing diabetes.

Insulin treatment for diabetes

People with type 1 diabetes are unable to produce enough insulin to regulate the glucose (sugar) levels within their blood, so they need to take insulin to manage their diabetes. Some people with type 2 diabetes and gestational diabetes (diabetes that develops during pregnancy) may also need insulin to control their blood sugar levels. There are a variety of types of insulin and ways to give it, including injections, pens and pumps. Your doctor and diabetes educator can recommend the most suitable type of insulin and delivery device for you.

Types of insulin

There are different types of insulin available to manage diabetes. These days, most types of insulin are synthetic (created in a laboratory), but there are some that are extracted from the pancreas of animals.

1. Types of insulin vary, according to:
2. how quickly they take effect;

3. how long their effect lasts; and
4. when they reach their peak, in terms of ability to lower blood-glucose levels.

Ultra-short-acting

Ultra-short-acting (also called very-short-acting or rapid-acting) insulin starts to work about 15 minutes after being injected, peaks after about 1-2 hours, and lasts for about 4-5 hours. This type of insulin is injected immediately before meal times and is also used in insulin pumps.

Types of ultra-short-acting insulin include:

- insulin glulisine (brand name Apidra);
- insulin lispro (Humalog); and
- insulin aspart (NovoRapid).

These are all synthetic copies (analogues) of human insulin and are clear in appearance.

Short-acting insulin

Short-acting insulin (insulin neutral) starts to work about half an hour after being injected, peaks from between 3 and 5 hours, and lasts for about 6-8 hours. Short-acting insulin is given 20-30 minutes before a meal. It is clear in appearance.

Types of short-acting neutral insulin include:

Actrapid and Humulin R (human short-acting insulins); and

Hypurin Neutral (short-acting insulin obtained from the pancreas of cattle – bovine insulin).

Intermediate acting insulin

Intermediate-acting insulin (isophane insulin) is cloudy in appearance. It starts to work 1-2 hours after being injected, peaks at 4-12 hours and lasts for 16-24 hours. Intermediate-acting insulin is usually given once or twice a day.

Types of intermediate-acting insulin include:

Humulin NPH and Protaphane (human isophane insulins); and

Hypurin Isophane (NPH) (bovine isophane insulin).

Intermediate-acting insulin is often used in conjunction with short-acting insulin.

Long lasting insuling

Long-acting insulin starts to work several hours after being injected and lasts for about 24 hours. It has no peak effect. Long-acting insulin is usually given once (or sometimes twice) daily, and should be given at the same time every day.

Types of long-acting insulin include:

insulin glargine (brand names Lantus, Toujeo); and

insulin detemir (brand name Levemir).

Both types of long-acting insulin are human insulin analogues (synthetic copies of human insulin) and are clear in appearance.

Mixed insulin

Mixed insulin (also called biphasic premixed or combination insulin) is a premixed combination of 2 different types of insulin.

Mixed insulin that contains short-acting neutral insulin and intermediate-acting isophane insulin include the following. (The numbers written after the brand name show the mix of the 2 types of insulin.)

Humulin 30/70 (which contains 30 per cent short-acting and 70 per cent intermediate-acting);

Mixtard 30/70; and

Mixtard 50/50.

The ultra-short acting insulins lispro and aspart are also available in a biphasic form. In this form some of the insulin is combined with a protein (protamine) to slow down its action.

Humalog Mix25 (insulin lispro);

Humalog Mix50 (insulin lispro); and NovoMix 30 (insulin aspart).

There is also a mixed insulin that contains a new type of ultra-long-acting basal insulin (insulin degludec) plus short-acting insulin aspart. This type of mixed insulin can be used in adults with diabetes. It is injected once (or sometimes twice) daily, with its effects lasting longer than 24 hours. The brand name is: Ryzodeg 70/30.

Mixed insulin is available in a pre-filled insulin pen and is particularly convenient for people who have poor eyesight or coordination, or who are unable to draw up insulin accurately from 2 different bottles of insulin.

Which insulin is best

The type of insulin that is best for you and the timing of doses will depend upon a range of different factors such as:

- the type of diabetes you have;

- your eating and exercise patterns; and
- your individual reaction to the different types of insulin available.

How is insulin taken

For people with , insulin can be given in one of the following ways.

Multiple daily injections: long-acting (or intermediate-acting) insulin is given once or twice a day as background insulin to maintain blood sugar levels – this is called a basal dose of insulin. Ultra-short-acting (or short-acting) insulin is also given just before meals and, if needed, to correct high blood sugar levels – these are called bolus doses of insulin.

Mixed insulin doses: combination (biphasic premixed) insulin is given once or twice daily.

Continuous insulin infusion: very short-acting insulin is given via an insulin pump. is usually treated with medicines and lifestyle changes to begin with, but most people with type 2 diabetes eventually also need to take insulin. Insulin treatment for type 2 diabetes usually starts with a once-daily basal dose of long-acting insulin. In people with very poorly controlled blood sugar levels, twice-daily basal doses, mixed insulin doses or multiple daily injections may be recommended.

Insulin delivery devices

Insulin is usually given using a needle and syringe, insulin pen injector or pump, and is injected into the layer of tissue just under your skin called the subcutaneous tissue. Insulin is absorbed fastest from the subcutaneous tissue of the abdomen, but can also be given to the thigh or buttocks.

Needles and syringe

A common way of administering insulin is with a needle and syringe. Syringes come in a range of capacities (1 mL, 0.5 mL or 0.3 mL) and with a range of needle types (different gauges — that is thicknesses — and lengths) attached. The needles have very fine points and special coatings to make injections relatively pain-free.

Your diabetes educator can help you select a syringe that suits the size of the insulin dose you take and that has your preferred needle type and needle size attached.

One of the main advantages of the syringe system is the variety of products available. Needles and syringes also make it easy to use a mixture of different types of insulin. However, some people find syringes daunting and not very convenient.

insulin pens

Insulin pen injectors (pen needles) are a convenient and discreet way of administering insulin. Many people find insulin pens easier to use than a needle and syringe.

Insulin pens have a built-in dial that allows you to determine the amount of insulin to be injected, a short needle at one end, and a plunger at the other. Some are disposable, and don't need to be assembled before use, while others have a replaceable insulin cartridge that needs to be inserted (much like a fountain pen cartridge).

Insulin pens are particularly useful if you take premixed insulin. They are also useful for people who have problems with their eyesight or problems such as arthritis of the hands that make it difficult to use a needle and syringe.

insulin pumps

Insulin pumps are small devices that run off batteries and are worn on your belt or in your pocket. They deliver insulin at a slow, continuous rate throughout the day, and also release larger quantities of insulin at meal times or when blood sugar levels are high.

The pump delivers the insulin via an infusion set (also called a giving set) – a thin tube ending in a cannula that is inserted under the skin of your abdomen and remains in place for several days (the cannula needs to be changed every 2-3 days).

The main advantage of insulin pumps is that they closely mimic the release of insulin by the pancreas. Pumps can help you achieve tighter blood glucose control and reduce the frequency of episodes of severe low blood sugar (hypoglycaemia). Many people with type 1 diabetes find that using insulin pumps improves their quality of life. However, using an insulin pump can be expensive.

When using an insulin pump, monitoring your blood glucose levels regularly (at least 4-6 times per day) is essential. Because pumps use ultra short-acting insulin, problems such as blockages can quickly lead to high blood sugar levels and . You should never disconnect from the pump for more than 2 hours without using an alternative method of delivering insulin, such as injections.

The latest types of insulin pumps can link with a continuous glucose monitoring system (CGMS) – a sensor device that is inserted under the skin and continuously measures glucose levels in the interstitial fluid (fluid in the body's tissues). CGMS devices can detect patterns in glucose levels during the day and night, providing insight on your overall glucose control.

Some CGMS devices can sound an alarm when glucose levels quickly become too high or too low, and when linked to an insulin pump can temporarily stop the pump delivering insulin if glucose levels fall too low.

Blood glucose checks with finger prick testing must still be done to determine insulin doses and also to calibrate the CGMS device.

Artificial pancreas device

Clinical trials are currently underway in Australia using an 'artificial pancreas' device to treat type 1 diabetes. The device is a closed-loop insulin pump system, where blood sugar levels are frequently monitored and then the appropriate amount of insulin is automatically delivered via an insulin pump.

Calculations to work out how much insulin to give are made using an algorithm (maths program) that mimics a healthy pancreas. The amount of insulin needed is adjusted based on your blood sugar levels and activities. This means that the person does not have to be constantly involved in monitoring their blood sugar levels and administering insulin. However, they can override the system if needed.

Treatment with this technology will hopefully allow people to have improved blood sugar control as well as greater flexibility and fewer injections.

Other delivery devices

Several other ways of delivering insulin have been investigated. These devices, which are not currently available or not commonly used in Australia, include the following.

Insulin inhalers, which deliver dry powdered insulin into the bloodstream via the lungs, have been used to deliver pre-mealtime insulin. Currently not available in Australia.

Insulin jet injectors work by sending a fine spray of insulin into the skin using a pressurised jet of air instead of a needle. However, jet injection isn't any less painful than administering insulin with a needle, and may cause bruising or altered absorption levels. Jet injectors also require frequent cleaning and maintenance. They are not commonly used.

Insulin sprays, either for the nose or mouth, and insulin pills are methods of insulin delivery that continue to be investigated.

Insulin patches are also currently under development, but it is difficult for insulin to be absorbed through the skin. The patch is designed to release insulin slowly and continuously.

Islet cell transplantation

Islet cell transplantation is a surgical procedure whereby islet cells from the pancreas of a human organ donor are injected into the liver of a recipient with type 1 diabetes. Islets (of Langerhans) contain beta cells, which secrete insulin. The transplanted cells begin to secrete insulin over time, and insulin doses may be reduced or, in some cases, insulin injections are no longer needed.

In Australia, islet cell transplantation is usually considered for people with type 1 diabetes who have difficulty keeping their blood sugar levels stable. It can help prevent episodes of low blood sugar (hypoglycaemia). The recipient needs to take immunosuppressive medicines for life to prevent rejection of the transplanted tissue.

Insulin plant for diabetes

Insulin Plant (Costus igneus)

Costus igneus a medicinal plant is a Magic Cure for Diabetes. Its leaves helps to build up insulin in the human body so it is commonly known as insulin plant in India This plant was grown in America and is becoming popular in India because of its medicinal chemicals. It is now accepted and used widely as an Ayurvedic medicinal herb. Consumption of the leaves are believed to lower blood glucose levels, and diabetics who consumed the leaves of this plant did report a fall in their blood glucose levels.

Insulin plant (Costus igneus) is native to Southeast Asia, especially on the Greater Sunda Islands in Indonesia. It is a relatively new entrant to Kerala and India. The plant is characterized by large fleshy looking leaves. The undersides of these large, smooth, dark green leaves have light purple shade. The leaves are spirally arranged around the stem, forming attractive, arching clumps arising from underground rootstocks.

The maximum height of these plants is about two feet. The flowers are orange in color and are beautiful, 1.5-inch diameter. Flowering occurs during the warm months. And they appear to be cone-like heads at the tips of branches. The flower petals are quite sweet and nutritious. It's a lower grower and makes a great ground cover. The long red flower spikes of Costus pulverulentus are unique to the family.

Costus igneus plant grows very quickly. Propagation of this plant is by stem cutting. It needs sunshine but it also grows in slightly shady areas. Costus does not have a problem with pests and diseases. Outdoor plants might be chewed by caterpillars, and in indoors plants might be affected by red spider mite.

Botanical name: - Costus igneus. Costus igneus common name is *Fiery Costus* or *Spiral Flag*, is a species of herbaceous plant in the Costaceae family. Insulin plant (Costus igneus) common name in Hindi is keukand and in Gujarati - pakarmula. In Marathi, Malayalam and Sanskrit is - pushkarmula and in Tamil is kostam.

Medicinal use

In Ayurvedic treatment diabetes patients are advised to chew down the Insulin plants leaves for a month. The patient has to take two leaves per day in the morning and evening for one week. The leaves must be chewed well before swallowing. After one week the patient should take one leaf each in the morning and evening. This dosage should be continued for 30 days. Allopathic doctors too recommend it and it is found to be effective in bringing blood sugar levels under completely under control. There is also dried and ground powder of the leaves now available in the market.

In Traditional Medicine it is also used to Promotes longevity, Treats rash, Reduces fever, Treats asthma , Treats bronchitis and to Eliminates intestinal worms. This plant is mentioned in the Kama Sutra as an ingredient in a cosmetic to be used on the eyelashes to increase sexual attractiveness.

Health Benefits Of Insulin Plant

Bogor Agricultural Institute (IPB) has conducted various researches related to this insulin plant. One of the researchers has proved that insulin leaves have a high fructose level. The excessive fructose is absorbed and filtered by the human digestive enzyme. This further normalizes the sugar level in the blood.2 Thus, it shows how crucial insulin leaves are for people suffering from diabetes. Following mentioned are some major health benefits of this leaf:

1. Curing Diabetes

As the name suggests, insulin leaves work best to cure diabetes by reducing the high sugar level inside the body.3 The increased sugar level in the blood is regulated by the amount of fructose present in the leaves.

Regular intake of insulin leaves can prevent chronic future health complications occurring from diabetes like organ failure and the free flow of nutrients in the body.

For treating diabetes prefer having a decoction prepared with insulin leaves. Boil few insulin leaves in water for good 10 minutes. Strain and drink this solution two times a day for good results.

2. Natural Pre-Biotic To Smooth Digestion

Insulin plant has various vitamins and complex components. The components work as good as the E-Coli bacteria. A good bacterial growth in the gut smoothens the functioning of the human digestive system and bring about the proper assimilation of the nutrients in the body.

Further, these leaves also have a high fructose level which helps in improving the colon function system. Thus, its consumption will also help to ease out the excretion process. Prefer chewing one to two leaves of insulin plant or having the decoction after having your meals for about a month.

3. Anti-Bacteria

Insulin plants have an anti-bacterial and anti-microbial activity. Methanolic extract of the plant shows maximum anti-bacterial activity against various gram-positive species like Bacillus cerus, Bacillus megaterium, Staphylococcusn aureus and various gram-negative strains like Pseudomonas aeruginosa, Escherichia coli, Klebsiella pneumoniae, and Salmonella typhimurium.5

So, if you have severe problems related to the kidneys or urination, try consuming these leaves regularly. The insulin leaves kill the bad bacteria inside the urinary pipe. Moreover, they automatically help in the smooth functioning of the excretory process and providing relief Yet, you still need to drink a lot of water to supplement it.

4. Natural Anti-Oxide

Oxidation is a natural chemical reaction which produces free radicals. These radicals trigger some dangerous illnesses like cancer and harm the skin beauty. This is why people are struggling to get free from such radicals.

A study showed that the insulin plant has moderate levels of antioxidative compounds in it.6 In the same study, it was found that the antioxidant activity of it was around 90.0% when compared with standard BHT (Butylated Hydroxy Toulene) (85%) at a concentration of 400 μg/ml.

It is the methanolic extracts of the leaves and rhizomes of insulin plants that have such high antioxidant activity. Thus, by regularly drinking insulin leaves, your body fights well and beat the oxidation process occurring inside the body cells.

5. Liver Illness Curing

Liver diseases occur as a result of fat deposition in the liver which further leads to other chronic illnesses. There are several vital components in the leaves of insulin plant that aid in breaking down the fatty acid deposition in the liver and thereby improving the liver functioning.

Thus, if you are struggling with a liver disease then start consuming this drink daily at least 2-3 times a day. This will help to erode away the poison stored inside the liver.

6. Kidneys Health

Leaves and rhizomes of insulin plant have a diuretic effect. They work to induced an increment in sodium and potassium clearance and thus giving regulating diuresis.7 With proper diuresis and a balanced excretory rate automatically, the kidney health improves.

If you are already suffering from kidney stones or kidney infections then start drinking the insulin leaves tea daily. This will help to ease out the functioning of the kidneys. When the kidneys start to malfunction then there is no way back and you will have to subject your body to dialysis.

7. Bladder Health

The insulin plant has compounds that are good diuretic and aid in bladder health too. It is very important to maintain the bladder health as if you do not take care of it, it may lead to infection. Thus, the insulin leaves potion can help in the urination process.

Prefer, drinking this potion before going to bed. It is because it will help in stimulating the bladder to work properly and eliminate healthily every morning.

8. Cancer Prevention

In a study done on the ethanolic extracts of one of the species of insulin plant it was found they have anti-proliferative and anti-cancer potential. Although, the study was done in in-vitro mammalian fibrosarcoma (HT-1080) cells.So, in this study, it was concluded the barks and leaves have anti-cancer properties against HT 29 and A549 cells. Consuming the insulin leaves regularly can prevent the growth of cancer cells inside the body.

9. Immunity

Insulin leaves have a natural anti-oxide character. This automatically enhances your body immune system by removing all the free radicals from the body. With a well-maintained immunity system, your body will remain healthy throughout. Start by drinking the insulin leaves and honey decoction regularly. Drink it at least twice a day if you have a weak immune system.

10. Reduction In Cholesterol

The insulin plant has a high amount of water water-soluble that slows down the absorption of glucose from the digestive system into the blood.9 Not only this it regulates the insulin production and sugar absorption ability of the body. This, in turn, brings about better assimilation and absorption of fats and thereby reducing the blood cholesterol levels in the body.

If you usually suffer from high cholesterol levels then you are at a higher risk of getting a heart attack, stroke, or cancer. Cholesterol is the biggest enemy of the body and thus it is important to avoid it. Start consuming insulin leaves every day which will help your body in breaking down the cholesterol from the food.

11. Cure For Asthma

Studies show that the plant has the ability to control the inflammation in the airways. Further, it also helps to soothe the muscles in the lungs that tend to tighten during an asthma attack. If you suffer from asthma then prefer consuming the insulin plant leaves to benefit you from asthma attacks.

12. Helps Alleviate Symptoms Of Bronchitis

Bronchitis occurs when the airways become narrow due to the inflammation of the airways and the excessive mucus present in them. The essential compounds present in the leaves of insulin plant work on to reduce the inflammation and thereby curing the condition. Daily consumption of tea infused with insulin leaves will help to reduce this inflammation and thus slowly and gradually cures Bronchitis.

How Insulin Plant Cures Diabetes

To answer that, first we need to understand What is Diabetes. Diabetes is a lifelong disease that occurs when our blood glucose, also called blood sugar level, is too high. Blood glucose is our main source of energy and comes from the food we eat. For our bodies to work properly we need to convert glucose or sugar into energy. Now Insulin, a hormone made by the pancreas, helps glucose get into our cells and converts glucose into energy. But sometimes our body doesn't make enough—or any—insulin or doesn't use insulin well. Glucose then stays in your blood and doesn't reach the cells which ultimately results in high blood glucose levels.

So to control Diabetes our body should produce and/or use enough insulin. And this is where Insulin Plant helps. This medicinal plant can help build up and strengthen the beta cells of the pancreas inside your body.

Moreover, it has a natural concentration of corosolic acid which shows a positive effect on blood sugar levels. Corosolic acid works in the process of metabolism and of the spread of glucose process like insulin that reduces the blood sugar levels by transporting the glucose into cells and out of the bloodstream. Thus its helps cure Diabetes. Diabetes can strike anyone, from any walk of life that requires daily self care. So let's take care of this condition with this amazing plant.

How To Recognize Insulin Plant

Insulin Plant is a perennial, upright, spreading plant reaching about two feet tall, with the tallest stems falling over and lying on the ground. Its leaves are simple, alternate, entire, oblong, evergreen, 4-8 inches in length with parallel venation. The leaves are large, smooth and dark green. The undersides of the leaves have light purple and are spirally arranged around stems, forming arching clumps arising from underground root-stocks. Flowers are orange in colour and are 1.5-inch in diameter. Flowering occurs during the warm months, appearing on cone-like heads at the tips of branches. This plant also produces inconspicuous fruits and they are not showy, less than 0.5 inch, and green-colored fruits.

From Where This Magical Herb Can Be Sourced

The southern part of India is abundant with this plant. Here, this plant is grown as ornamental plant in gardens and is quite available. This plant is also being cultivated in Kashmir and the Himalayan regions for its root. The other parts of the world where this plant is available is South and Central America. In-fact this is the native place of this plant. In this region it is commonly known as Fiery Costus or Step Ladder or Spiral Flag or Insulin Plant.

Different Names Of Insulin Plant

Insulin Plant- A Magic Cure For Diabetes

Insulin Plant in India is known in different names in different states. Let's see the local names of the plant in different languages.

Bengali- Piasal

Hindi- Banda or Boja sal or Peisar or Jarul or Keukand

Kannada- Kampu Honne

Malayalam- Honne or Vengai

Tamil- Koslam

Sankrit- Asana

Marathi- Honi

Oriya- Vengis

Telegu- Peddavesiga

Gujrati- Pakarmula

Urdu- Bijasar

How to use Insulin plant to cure diabetes – DIY
Fiery costus or spiral flag, is a herbal plant from costaceae family native of Brazil. In India, it is known as "Insulin plant" because of its use in Ayurveda and siddha

medicine to treat diabetes (1). The leaves of the plant are dark green and fleshy. The plant grows up to a height of about two feet with a number of broad lengthy leaves forming around the stem like a spiral.

Nutrition information

The plant is mainly used for its anti-diabetic properties even though it contains many other medicinal properties. There are studies that suggest the usage of the plant in the treatment of Ascaris, asthma, and bronchitis.

The study on the contents of the insulin plant and its application in the modern medical field is in initial stages only. Only during recent years some authenticated studies and the observations have been revealed.

How to make insulin leaves raita

The recipe here is simple and is a healthy way to consume the leaves of insulin plant. You can consume this raita daily as accompaniment for rice, bread and roti.

Servings Prep Time

2 people 10 minutes

Ingredients

- 8 leaves Insulin leaves
- 1 cup Homemade yogurt / curd
- 1 teaspoon Pepper
- 1/2 teaspoon Salt

Instructions

The ingredients required for making insulin leaves raita are shown below. If you are unable to prepare yogurt at home, you can buy plain yogurt and use that.

Chop the insulin leaves using a knife or a pair of scissors. The leaves are crunchy in texture and can be chopped well.

Keep the chopped leaves aside. These leaves taste mildly sour and are suitable for making raita.

Add the chopped leaves to yogurt. Use fresh yogurt for making raita.

Mix well.

Add a teaspoon of ground pepper and a pinch of salt to the yogurt.

Mix all the ingredients together.

The raita is now done. You can also refrigerate it for a while and serve it chilled.

Recipe Notes

Tips for growing insulin plant:

This plant needs sun shine to grow. It can be grown in fields as well as in home gardens where adequate sun shine is available. It is a perennial plant. The stem cuttings are planted and grown. No seed is required.

The leaves are sweet and sour and you can consume it raw.

When can you see results?

It is established that results of regular consumption of insulin plant can be seen only after fifteen days of consumption.

Research evidence

Evidence 1

Ethanolic extract of Costus igneus (insulin plant) has the ability to conduct antidiabetic effect. The study and research has proved that the diabetes level has reduced when tested in diabetic rats. This particular study had brought the plant to the notice of many scientists who are carrying researches in fining treatment options for diabetes mellitus from Costus igneus leaves.

Evidence 2

Studies show that when the insulin leaves from the insulin plant (Costus igeus) are consumed regularly, it reduces the fasting blood sugar level and postprandial blood sugar levels. This study has brought down the sugar levels to normal when tested in dexamethasone-induced hyperglycemia rats.

These research evidence show that the regular consumption of the plant leaves and its extract can help you reduce blood sugar levels effectively. The extract of the leaves are available in powder form which can be used in making tea or can be mixed in warm water and consumed.

How To Consume Insulin Plant To Cure Diabetes-

Diabetes can strike anyone, from any walk of life that requires daily self care. So let's take care of this condition with this amazing plant. There are mainly three ways in which insulin plant can be consumed to cure diabetes. Let's see below the different ways...

1. Chewing

If your blood sugar level is too high i-e above 200 then

Chew two leaves in the morning and two leaves in the evening for first week

From the second week one leaf in the morning and one in the evening.

This dosage should be continued for 30 days. The leaves of Insulin plant must be chewed well before swallowing. After chewing the leaves have some water.

2. Insulin Plant Tea

Insulin plant tea is also effective in reducing diabetes.

Simply make a decoction by pounding one leaf and boiling it in water till it reduces in half.

Consume this water daily in the morning and night.

3. Insulin Plant Powder

The third way is insulin plant powder.

Take out some leaves from the plant and dry them in the shade

Then grind them and make a fine powder.

Consume ½ teaspoon of insulin plant powder every day

Note-You can also buy insulin plant powder from the market but making the powder by yourself will help you get the maximum benefits as no extra artificial compound will be present in the powder.

Precaution

Consumption of insulin plant without knowing the proper dosage may adversely affect your health.

Above dosages are in general. One should take suggestions from medical supervisor before consuming it.

Pregnant and lactating women should avoid consuming this plant.

How To Make Insulin Leaves Steeping

1. Pick ten plus insulin leaves. Cut them into small slices and wash them under flowing water.

2. Dry these leaves under the sun. You may check the dried leaves by squeezing them.

3. The dried leaves are ready to be steeped now. Take a cup of water and let it boil. Once it starts to boil pour it into the glass wherein you have already placed some dried insulin leaves.

4. Wait a moment until the water in the glass turns brown.

5. You may add honey to this mixture for a better taste. Start drinking this regularly for best results.

How To Make Tea Of Insulin Leaves

Insulin Leaves Steeping for making tea

Insulin Leaves Steeping for making tea

Pick 5-7 slices of fresh insulin leaves from the tree.

Wash under the flowing water and then let it dry out for a moment.

Prepare a pot to boil 3-5 cups of water.

Wait a moment until the water starts to boil. Then put the leaves into the water. Let the water boil until it reduces only to about one cup.

Switch off the stove and filter the insulin leaves before pouring it into the cup. You may add some honey for taste purposes.

Drink regularly at least once a day for best results.

Final Talk

Now, you know the array of health benefits of insulin plant and the ways to take it. If you wish you can start consuming it from today itself to improve your health. However, if you face any issue after consuming it immediately discontinue the use and consult a doctor if required.

Printed in Dunstable, United Kingdom

72142818R00037